Defeating Mental Illness

Defeating Mental Illness

by
Nick Griemsmann

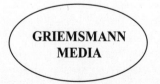

GRIEMSMANN
MEDIA

Defeating Mental Illness by Nick Griemsmann
Published by Griemsmann Media
P.O. Box 60065
Phoenix, Arizona 85082
www.GriemsmannMedia.com

Visit the author's website: www.TheFathersFriends.org

Scripture Quotations

King James Bible, public domain

New King James Version of the Bible. Copyright 1979, 1980, 1982 by Thomas Nelson, Inc., publishers.

KJ3 Literal Translation Bible, First Edition, Copyright © 2006 Jay P. Green, Sr.

Copyright © 2013 by Nick Griemsmann

First Edition: July 2013
Printed in the United States of America
ISBN: 978-1-62847-157-1

CONTENTS

FORWARD

Millions and millions of people struggle with mental illness and this book is specifically dedicated to those hurting individuals. My prayer is that this book helps someone out there find relief from the torment of mental illness.

Please know that I, Nick Griemsmann, am not a professional (or licensed) counselor, psychiatrist, or any other medically trained person. I am just someone who cares about the mentally ill and really want to help people who are on their recovery journey.

This book was written to inform the reader about my personal testimony of overcoming schizophrenia and is meant to encourage, not to put down anyone. The things written in this book are to try to help people and not meant to judge or offend any individual or group of people. I deeply care for every person and truly believe that there is great hope for people to fully recover from all types of mental illnesses.

I am personally trying my best to help those people out there that are seeking freedom. This book was written out of love and I sincerely hope it sheds some light on you and in turn gives you and others hope for freedom from mental illness.

God bless you and your family!

Nick Griemsmann

This book is dedicated to every person who is tormented by a mental illness. God has not forgotten you.

CHAPTER 1
Batons, Airports and Hollywood

"It is incurable." said the psychiatrist to my mother and me. It was the fall of 2003 and we were sitting in a county behavioral health clinic in Phoenix, Arizona. "Incurable?" my mother said back to her. The psychiatrist was in her early 70's, very depressed looking and staunch in her reply back to my mother, "Yes, paranoid schizophrenia is an incurable mental illness. Your son will always have to take the prescribed medications, collect (government) disability, either live with you or in a group home, never be able to hold down a job and will definitely not ever be able to have a family of his own." She went on to say, "And sometimes with these types of cases, after ten or so years the patient might go into a catatonic like state which is kind of like being what we would call - a vegetable."

My mother's mouth dropped open as she hopelessly looked over at me, her 23 year old son who could barely speak because the "voices" had taken over almost his entire mind. She grabbed my hand and said, "Nick, it's going to be alright!"

The full effect of what that doctor told us that day didn't really hit me until a few weeks later. As I sat on the couch in my mother's home (that's where I was living at the time), all at once I realized that a doctor had diagnosed me with an "incurable" mental illness and that I was never (so I thought) going to get any better.

I believed the doctor's opinion for over six months, until I chose to do something about it; fight back!

This book is written to help people out there that struggle with or who know someone who struggles with what the doctors have labeled a "mental illness". In some countries around the globe, instead of labeling someone with a mental illness, they just say the person is experiencing "madness" or is "mad". My prayer is that this book helps you find hope for recovery.

I was diagnosed schizophrenic in my early twenties. To be exact, it was the week before my 23rd birthday. Like most kids, I grew up in a pretty normal non-religious household. My parents divorced when I was eight years old and my dad wasn't around much after that so I learned a lot about being a man from watching television and from my older brother.

Fast forward to the late 1990's; I ended up dropping out of high school in 10th grade because I had a bad marijuana and alcohol addiction. By the time I was 19 years old; I was a bartender and was struggling through community college. A nightclub opened up down the street from where I was working, and at 21 years old I was bartending at a fancy nightclub in upscale Scottsdale, Arizona. I was mingling with rich people, doing a lot of drugs, drinking heavily and completely without any real direction for my life.

As a nightclub bartender, I started to feel really convicted for pouring drinks for people who I knew were going to drive home drunk. Also, I felt convicted for being part of a place where people who I knew were married, were trying to "hook up" with other people in the nightclub.

This conviction for my lifestyle started leading me to seeking out God. It started with me occasionally watching religious broadcasts on television and then I eventually bought a Bible. I remember that I used to hide the Bible underneath my bathroom counter in my apartment because I was afraid my roommates would think I was crazy for reading it. I remember always feeling "pulled" in my heart towards Jesus. The problem was; I didn't know how to find release from all the conviction that I felt for my party lifestyle. It seemed as though the feeling of guilt just kept piling up on top of me, with no relief. You kind of might feel like that today. You might feel as if your lifestyle isn't right and you have maybe felt convicted in your heart about it. Let me tell you something wonderful; God is nearer then you think and He cares about you. In reality, God literally is just a prayer away.

One day, I decided to call a Christian prayer line. The lady on the phone asked me, "Are you saved?" I didn't understand what she meant because it seemed to me that different denominations and religions all had a different take on what "saved" really meant. She then asked me to pray a prayer with her and led me in a repentance prayer to God and I asked Jesus Christ to save me and wash me in His blood.

At first, I was just saying the prayer because I felt like I had to because the lady was kind of pushy, but I am so glad she led me in that prayer that day. Immediately, as a said the name of Jesus, I could feel the Holy Spirit rush over me and clean my entire soul from sin. It was amazing and I will never forget it! I got saved that day at the age of 22. With that one simple prayer of faith, I was instantly delivered from the party lifestyle, drinking and drugs.

During this time in my life, I was browsing the Internet for churches that preached the truth. I happened to fall on a website for a man who claimed to be one of the final Two Witnesses mentioned in the Book of Revelation. Of course, he was not one of the Two Witnesses, but I being so young in the knowledge of God's word, totally "fell for it".

On his website, it said that his church provided all the things necessary for life (clothing, food, shelter, etc) to all those who truly wanted to serve the Lord with all of their heart, soul, mind and strength. Obviously, I just had gotten saved from a life of sin and I was so thankful that all I wanted to do was serve Jesus for the rest of my life. I decided to move away from my family and friends and live at one of his church compounds to "serve the Lord". The compound where I ended up living was in Arkansas.

Long story short; I ended up moving into the church and everything seemed "ok" at first. But now that I look back, there were some red flags for me that I was in a cult. I believe that I overlooked them because I was so excited to be away from all my drinking buddies back in Phoenix. Within a month or so, the church people told me that my family was of the devil and that I was not to have anymore phone contact with them. They told me once in a while I could send letters, but that was pretty much it. I thought this was weird, but by this point I thought I had found the "one true church" and believed that I was being taught by one of the last day prophets. But I would soon find out that it was all a big lie.

At the church compound, whenever anyone would get in trouble or someone "told on" you for doing something against the prophet's commands, the person would get a cassette tape from the church office. For instance, I wore a pair of shorts into the church sanctuary and they said that I was sinning against the Lord and that I could burn in hell for not listening to the commands of the prophet. I was scared! I was moved by fear to obey whatever they told me were his commands.

The cassette tapes given to members were what I refer to as "rebuking cassettes". One time I saw a man in the apartment house that I was staying at get one of these tapes from the leader and he was shaking in horror. He played the tape and the pastor was yelling at him telling him he was going to burn in hell if he didn't repent, follow his commands, etc. The poor man was frightened out of his mind and I was too!

Along with these "rebuking cassettes" that we would receive, it was mandatory to go to church service every night at about 7:00pm. During these redundant services, we would do three songs for worship, listen to short testimonies, an older person in the church would come up and share from the Bible (usually about hell) and then they would play the nightly church service cassette tape from the leader or watch conspiracy theory videos on a television set. When we did have to listen to the leader preach from one of his cassettes, it was almost always on hell fire and brimstone which freaked me out so much! I was literally in fear and torment everyday because I thought God was this mean old man in the sky that wanted to burn everyone alive in hell. I never did see or meet the leader of the cult, he wasn't even at the church facility, but was in a different location living with a bunch of little girls as his wives. Crazy, huh? Of course, I didn't know this until he was arrested after I was out of the cult (I left the cult in Dec. 2003) and everything was on the news in 2009. He currently is now in federal prison serving a 175 year sentence for child molestation.

About five months into being at the cult and filled with tons of fear and torment about hell, I started hearing voices in my mind that I thought were angels or the Holy Spirit. The voices eventually had me run off during a ministry trip to Nashville, Tennessee where they found me screaming in the International Airport there. What happened that day was that the voices told me to run off from the ministry trip (we used to drive around city to city putting anti-government and hellfire tracts on cars parked in large parking lots) so one night I ran out of the hotel room and the next day found myself homeless (and hearing voices) walking by a field by the Nashville International Airport.

I remember lying in the grass afraid that because I had left the cult (they told me if someone ever left their "one true church" that it meant they had lost their salvation and had blasphemed the Holy Spirit) that I would never be able to be saved again.

I was listening to the voices in my mind and I eventually went into the airport baggage claim area to get a drink of water and to use the restroom. Inside the airport, the voices started telling me to get on my knees in the baggage claim area, close my eyes, and start praying to God really loud for everyone to hear. The voices told me if I did what they told me to do then God would "translate" me out of the airport and to somewhere else to preach.

So, that's what I did, I walked right out in the middle of the baggage claim area (there was about 200-300 people around me) and I dropped to my knees, closed my eyes, and started screaming to God in prayer! That was until the airport police arrived - Thunk! Pow! Ouch!

After getting yelled at to stop (I wouldn't stop) I got hit by them and it really hurt. I hit the floor still screaming to God (I thought the louder I screamed to God the faster He would come and translate me) and they then hog tied me and dragged me out of the airport. Talk about a wild scene at the airport!

After trying to talk with me, they noticed that I was extremely dehydrated and in need of mental health treatment. I ended up being locked up in one of Nashville mental hospitals for a couple of weeks for observation. I spent my 23rd birthday in a mental hospital. How sad is that, huh?

After being finished with the observation time, I was released and put on a bus back to Phoenix, Arizona. Once I got home, my family could tell that I had been brainwashed by the cult. All I could talk about was the Bible and that people were going to go to hell unless they repented and joined the one true church in Arkansas. There was nothing they could do for me. My mother was frightened and my other family members pretty much just stayed away from me.

Somehow I ended up on a bus back to the cult after spending about one month with my family and taking medications for paranoid schizophrenia. This time, I went to the cult outpost over by Hollywood, California instead of the outpost in Arkansas. While I was at the compound in California, I didn't take the prescribed medications that I received in Phoenix. This was because I didn't believe that I had a mental illness and also at the cult they said I couldn't take any medications. Over a course of about two weeks at the cult in California without my medications, I started having really horrible hallucinations, hearing even louder voices, and doing some pretty weird stuff. So weird, that one evening the church leaders told me to grab all of my belongings because they said, "You are going to go street preaching." I grabbed all of my belongings and jumped into their van really excited to have the chance to tell people about Jesus!

Instead, these men from the church stopped off at a fast food restaurant, walked me in, and bought me a sub sandwich. I put my head down to take a bite of my sandwich and the two men were gone. I was scared out of my mind. I thought I had blasphemed the Holy Spirit and had lost my salvation – again! I walked outside to look for the men from the church but I couldn't find a trace of them. The voices then came to me and they told me to close my eyes and said if I opened them up I would go immediately to hell. So, I listened to the voices and did everything they said. You have to remember that I was a young man who really loved Jesus and wanted to serve Him. I actually thought God was speaking to me in my head outside of that restaurant that night. It sounds almost too unbelievable, huh?

Not too much longer after leaving the fast food place, I found a bus stop on the sidewalk and fell asleep on it. I woke up with the sun rising. I was so scared. I thought that I had lost my salvation. What was I to do? Where could I go? The church had kicked me out and they were the only one true church, so I thought. The voices came talking to me again as I woke up that morning. I still remember it like it was yesterday. They said, "Jesus Christ is coming back to judge the world right now, look up and see." So, I looked up at the sun and it was coming through the clouds and I had a hallucination that it was Jesus riding a white horse coming to judge the world. Then the voices said, "You have to show the world that you are not ashamed of Jesus Christ." I said back to them, "I am not ashamed of Jesus, I love Him!" Then the voices replied, "Then take off all of your clothes and show the world that you are not ashamed of Jesus!"

So, yes, that's what I did. On a street corner in Hollywood, California in 2003, only six months after knowing Jesus as my Lord and Savior, I took off all of my clothes in public and walked down the street completely naked. An ambulance came and they took me to the Emergency Room and I eventually ended up in another psyche hospital for observation.

There is more to this story, but I just wanted to share a little bit of it in this book with you so that you can be encouraged that the person writing this book about defeating mental illness has dealt with some pretty traumatic experiences and that I understand a lot about what you and/or your loved one(s) are going through.

I used to have lots of scary hallucinations. Believe it or not, the radio and television would talk directly to me. At one point, my neighbor's television set felt connected to my brain waves! I also had so much anxiety inside of my stomach and mind that I couldn't even take my dog for a walk outside. I was so scared! I even thought the President of the USA had me under surveillance at one point in my life. I had an alien type man appear next to me one time and he started conversing with me. I had lots of different people talk to me that weren't really even there. I had people who I thought were "angels" appear to me and some other really weird things that most people would never believe. You could say I was in a pretty hopeless situation in my early twenties.

There are a lot of other things that I could tell you about with my hallucinations and trips to and from over six different psychiatric wards across four states (Tennessee, California, Arizona and Oklahoma), but this book is not my personal testimony book; it is a book on encouraging you in your recovery from mental illness.

Believe it or not, during and after my schizophrenia recovery, I worked in the behavioral health field in

Phoenix, Arizona. I used my story of hope for recovery to help many mentally ill individuals. As an Administrator for a behavioral health company, I used my experience to impart knowledge and wisdom in the design of classes, groups and other things to help the mentally ill throughout the community. I also was invited to speak at conferences and events to share my recovery story with others. I have been interviewed both on video and for articles written by people in the behavioral health field from different parts of the country.

In writing this book, I am not only coming from experience with my own personal struggles with mental illness but also incorporating my years of working in the behavioral health field and some of my Christian ministry experience to help empower you in your recovery journey.

In the next few chapters, I am going to go over the below key points. I sincerely hope this book helps you in some way, shape or form. God bless you as you continue to read on with an open heart and mind.

KEY POINTS

- What is a mental illness and where could it actually come from?
- Some steps that I took that could help you in your own recovery from mental illness.
- How I believe that you can minister whole person freedom to yourself and others.
- Breaking the lies wrapped inside the mind.

CHAPTER 2
What Would Jesus Do?

The term mental illness is a term most (not all) people
use to describe someone who suffers from a disorder of
the mind. Some of the terms you might have heard before
are Bipolar Disorder, Clinical Depression, Paranoid
Schizophrenia, Schizoaffective Disorder, Post Traumatic
Stress Disorder (PTSD), Multiple Personality Disorder
(MPD), Obsessive Compulsive Disorder (OCD), General
Anxiety Disorder (GED), etc.

I believe most of these illnesses get their labels from the
"symptoms" that the person manifests in their life. For
instance, if you are bipolar, it is usually because you go
from a high-high in your personality and actions to a
low-low, hence the term bipolar. If you are
schizophrenic, it is usually because they say that you
have a distorted reality, voices in the mind and/or have
visual or audio hallucinations. Make sense?

Most of these diagnoses are because of what the doctors
will tell you are "chemical imbalances" in the brain.
Because of these chemical imbalances they administer
psychiatric medications to help "stabilize" the person.
According to almost all in the medical field, mental
illness is pretty much 100% incurable. Most doctors will
say that even though these illnesses are incurable, they
are manageable illnesses. Meaning; the doctors tell
people that they will have these illnesses for the rest of
their lives and basically give them no hope for complete
recovery.

I still remember one time I was giving my recovery story in a behavioral health care setting and after I was finished speaking a psychiatrist raised her hand to what I thought was to ask me a question but instead seemed upset. This doctor told me (and everyone else in attendance) that fully recovering from schizophrenia was impossible because it was an incurable mental illness. She was trying to say that I was misdiagnosed and never really had schizophrenia. I had to let her know that I had hundreds of pages of medical records (I still do) indicating that many different doctors all diagnosed me the same thing - schizophrenic. She wasn't realizing this one thing though; I had Jesus Christ on my side. He was my healer and deliverer. He healed me of mental illness and He can heal you too!

So, where does mental illness come from? I am not a doctor or medical professional so I can't answer that question in a medical sense, but I can try to answer it in a biblical sense. I figure you want the truth here, correct? This might be kind of scary for you, but I have to tell the truth here because I am trying to help someone out there.

In my own experience, it was revealed to me that I had evil spirits (yes, demons) attached to my brain somehow (I don't really know exactly how that all works) and through the word of God I was set free from all of the demons causing mental illness and torment.

This might be the first time that you have ever heard of mental illness possibly being caused by evil spirits, or what are called demons, but I can tell you that through years of ministry and also working in the behavioral health field, that this is a true statement. Let me say this though, <u>not all mental illness is caused by evil spirits,</u> some illnesses are caused by other issues not related to demons.

In this book, I want to show you some truths that I personally learned to help you in your recovery from mental illness.

When I was struggling with schizophrenia, my mother used to go on the Internet and search for resource after resource to try to help me with my illness. I still remember every night she would sit on the computer looking at websites and reading articles about schizophrenia cures and other things. She had me eating fish a lot because that was supposed to help with my brain chemistry somehow. I don't know if that really worked but I do want to put a "plug" in for my mother in this book. Thank you mother for being so strong and standing by me during the toughest times in my entire life, I love you!

Over many years, I have talked to many people about mental illness. Almost everybody believes that mental illness is caused strictly by a chemical imbalance. Even most Christians dismiss that demons could be attached to a brain possibly causing a chemical imbalance. But sad to say, a lot of people who believe this way are usually not completely free themselves. I am free from mental illness! I used to have to take over eight medications per day and every two weeks I had to go to my behavioral health care clinic to receive a medication shot in my rear end. It was so very shameful to have to pull my pants down and get a shot from a nurse every two weeks for my mental illness. But I am glad I went through what I did so I can have an opportunity to help someone else see the light at the end of the tunnel.

You may ask, "Well, what about children with mental illnesses, they can't have evil spirits, can they?" And the answer to that is, "Yes, they can." Once again though, not all mental illness is caused by demons. But if you look at what Jesus did in the Gospels it says that He not only cast demons out of adults but also out of young children. Please read the two verses

below. Notice that in the first passage it was a "young boy" and in the second passage it was a "young girl" who Jesus cast demons out of.

Matthew 17:14-18
And when they had come to the multitude, a man came to Him, kneeling down to Him and saying, "Lord, have mercy on my son, for he is an epileptic and suffers severely; for he often falls into the fire and often into the water. So I brought him to Your disciples, but they could not cure him." Then Jesus answered and said, "O faithless and perverse generation, how long shall I be with you? How long shall I bear with you? Bring him here to Me." And Jesus rebuked the demon, and it came out of him; and the child was cured from that very hour.

Mark 17:25-30
For a woman whose young daughter had an unclean spirit heard about Him, and she came and fell at His feet. The woman was a Greek, a Syro-Phoenician by birth,

*and she kept asking Him to cast the demon out of her
daughter. But Jesus said to her, "Let the children be
filled first, for it is not good to take the children's bread
and throw it to the little dogs." And she answered and
said to Him, "Yes, Lord, yet even the little dogs under the
table eat from the children's crumbs." Then He said to
her, "For this saying go your way; the demon has gone
out of your daughter." And when she had come to her
house, she found the demon gone out, and her daughter
lying on the bed.*

From my experience, I have come to the conclusion that
some kids who have been diagnosed with a mental illness
could have gotten the illness from a generational curse,
from being neglected, abused, molested, or even from
watching/listening to bad things in the media.

Believe it or not, many kids nowadays struggle with
anxiety because they have grown up watching things they
probably shouldn't have. Did you know that evil spirits
can come through movies and television with
fear/violence in them as well as soft pornography type
films that kids might watch? Other ways can include
playing really "dark" video games and the
cursing/swearing in music that kids listen to on their MP3
players. Does this kind of make sense to you? Garbage
in, garbage out, the more perversion, violence and
darkness children take in, the more problems they could
eventually have in their lives as they grow older.

I know this might be new to you, but please keep reading
with an open heart and mind because I believe this book
could possibly help you. I have found that most adult

mental illnesses are caused by past abuse, trauma, alcohol/drug use, etc. Many of our soldiers get Post Traumatic Stress Disorder (PTSD) because of the horrific experiences during times of war. Other people get mental illnesses because of abuse from a spouse, spiritual abuse from a church (like I did), childhood trauma, being raped/molested, etc. These types of "causes" are all pretty much tied to something that you might find interesting – sin.

For instance, a child is abused by their family member. This is a sin that lets in evil spirits to torment that child with memories, pain, etc. Somehow (I don't know exactly how) the child gets wounded in their soul/heart which can open up a door for evil spirits to possibly cause a mental illness and to torment the hurt child. Many times the mental illness won't manifest until later on in the child's life. Think of it this way; a plant seed being planted and eventually that evil seed becomes a large evil tree (the tree representing the mental illness or a possible physical disease later on in life). It takes a while for the seed to become a large tree, but it eventually grows up. Same way to look at how demons get into someone's life and eventually could lead them to having a mental illness or physical illness later on down the road. So, sometimes a mental illness that manifests in an older adult could be connected to something that happened when they were a young child. Make sense?

If a soldier sees his comrades blown up from a hand grenade attack, this could allow a demon of fear/trauma to come into the soldier's mind and cause a mental illness later on in his/her life.

A person could do crack cocaine and destroy their brain cells and allow demons of addiction into their brain that could manifest as a mental illness. An abused wife that gets verbally destroyed by her husband and in turn hates herself, has thoughts of suicide, depression, etc, which could lead to evil spirits entering the thoughts of the person and manifesting a mental illness. A child beat up at school by a bully turns to inner rage/anger (both could be demons) and eventually could get diagnosed with some sort of mental illness. The list goes on and on…

The point I am trying to get you to see is that most mental illness cases can be linked to some sort of sin or spiritual problem in the individual's past or present. What about you? How was your childhood? How has your life gone so far? Don't worry, there is hope!

I'M IN THE FIRES OF HELL

I met a person struggling with a mental illness a while back. She was a forty something year old woman. She reported to me that she had three kids that were living with her ex-husband. She said that her ex-husband used to beat her and verbally abuse her every day. She said that she was a normal teenage girl and at the age of 19 she began using marijuana as a party drug. She met her husband and they had three children together.

Within several years of verbal and physical abuse from her husband, she stared having hallucinations and was diagnosed mentally ill. I don't know exactly what she was diagnosed with but I am guessing she might have been struggling with schizophrenia. This is the interesting part; this lady would sit in groups/classes and complain of "pain" underneath her skin.

When I talked to her about the pain she said that God had sent her to hell and even though she lived on earth she actually was in a spiritual hell and that fire lived underneath her skin as hot as the real fires of hell. She said that it hurt so bad and no doctor could diagnose it and that everyone thought that she was making up the story, but to her it was 100% real. She believed that she had fire underneath her skin because she could honestly feel it! This horrible feeling had lasted for many years and she couldn't get away from it. It had led her to sheer hopelessness to where she thought about suicide almost every day. She could never get any relief from the torment. You might not have these same types of symptoms but maybe something similar. There is hope for you!

One day, I had a conversation with the lady about God. I was very gentle in my approach and asked her about her spiritual life. She said that she was saved (surrendered her heart/life to Jesus) as a young girl and over the course of several years she had been prayed over by many pastors and couldn't be free from the flames of hell. She said that Jesus didn't hear her prayers anymore because she had lost her salvation because she was evil. I talked with her and tried to explain the truth that she didn't lose her salvation because God loves her and forgives her.

I also talked with her about some of the other lies she believed but didn't get too far with her. I tried to help her but that day she was not in a place of discussion. Soon after that conversation I never saw her again at the facility. I hope God someday delivers her from the lies and the torment that she reported to me. It broke my heart to see this woman tormented like she was. There are thousands and thousands of people just like her in the world.

Do you see how the woman's whole mental illness could have possibly been caused by evil spirits lying to her? Do you see how through her drug use and the abuse from her husband the demons could have attached to her brain and thought patterns? Could it be that through sin (her own and her husband's) this woman was now being tormented by demons?

What I have found is that after the demons get in the mind of an individual, they torment them with lies. If the person keeps believing the lies, they could then actually start having hallucinations ie: seeing things others don't see, hearing voices, feeling bugs inside of them, living in paranoia, being in flames of hell, etc. These things could actually all be caused by demons. My question for you; after reading some of this book already, do you believe that some mental illness "symptoms" could possibly be caused by demons?

CHAPTER 3
Some Steps That Helped Me

Let's say that you believe that demons are causing your
mental illness. How can you be set free? That's what you
want, right; the steps to freedom? I am sorry, but I don't
have all the answers and I can't tell you exactly what to
do to be set free. This is because I don't know everything
about mental illness and I am surely not God. God has
different ways of healing His children. Some people
receive instant miracles and others slowly recover.
Everybody's situation is a bit different. But what I can do
is give you some steps that I used personally to be set
free from schizophrenia and maybe they will help you (or
someone you know) be set free as well.

STEP #1
Becoming a disciple of Jesus Christ

Luke 9:23
*Then He said to them all, "If anyone desires to come
after Me, let him deny himself, and take up his cross
daily, and follow Me."*

That was my first step. I decided (in my heart) to become
a disciple of Jesus Christ. Not a religious person, but to
pursue a personal relationship with God. I chose to read
Jesus' words, believe them and do them. It wasn't always
easy, but I did (and still do) my best to put Jesus first in
my life and circumstances. If you haven't been born
again or what we call "saved" yet and would like to start
a personal relationship with Jesus Christ, you can pray a

prayer similar to the prayer below. I believe if you really want to be saved right now, you can pray to God and He will meet you right now. He cares about you!

SAMPLE PRAYER

"Dear God, I come to You today and I choose to confess all of my sins to You. I ask that You come and touch my heart and help me repent of every sin in my life. I confess with my mouth Jesus Christ is Lord and believe in my heart that God raised Him from the dead. I ask that You, Jesus, wash my sins in Your precious blood and save my soul right now. Please fill me with your Holy Spirit, Jesus. I choose in my heart to become a disciple of Jesus Christ today. I pray this from my heart to God the Father in the name of Jesus Christ of Nazareth, amen."

If you truly believe you were just saved, congratulations!

Moving on with becoming a disciple of Jesus Christ; so, as I daily surrendered my heart to Jesus, I learned how to pray. That was one of my best tools that I learned how to use – prayer. After I was less fearful of churches after getting out of the cult in Arkansas, I found a good Spirit-filled church by my mother's home where I would go for services. I also learned to worship God. I recommend anyone struggling with mental illness to find a good place of worship so you can feel the presence of the Holy Spirit and be healed by Him inside and out.

As I attended this particular church, I was invited to some prayer meetings. I started to learn how to pray. Prayer to me was my life line to God. I couldn't go a day without praying. At first, I started praying for only one minute per night because of the torment and voices in my mind. But after I started out small with my prayer life; I eventually could spend one to two hours per night in prayer to God. Through the discipline of prayer, I grew closer to Jesus and then one day He showed up for me in a huge way – deliverance!

STEP #2
Realizing your authority

When I was mentally ill, my mother called all the churches in our area and asked for help with her schizophrenic son and most churches said that they didn't know how to help me or that they didn't believe in demons or deliverance. When I finally learned that I could actually get deliverance from the demons tormenting my mind, I was so happy!

I first received a book from a lady that I met at my local church about deliverance. I also went on the Internet and read about deliverance as well as talked with some Christians about it. I couldn't believe it; I could actually cast demons out of myself. What a revelation! What a miracle! What hope I had!

So, one day, I started walking around my mother's pool out back of her house. I was walking back and forth, round and round, praying to Jesus to help me cast out my demons. I started commanding satan to come out and after about one hour of telling the demons to come out, I felt a huge demon fly out of my head. It left with so much force that I fell to the ground. I was ecstatic! I just cast out my first demon and I finally knew that I was on my way to total freedom!

I know this all might be new to you and might sound a little crazy, but please keep reading because I believe this book could possibly help you or someone you love.

STEP #3
The road of repentance

Another thing that went along with my prayer life and deliverance was repentance. I didn't really understand repentance at the time, but now that I look back that's what I was kind of doing all along. I call it "dealing with my junk". That's what I believe everyone has to do – deal with your junk!

What type of "junk" do you have in your life? Are you living with your girlfriend/boyfriend before marriage? Do you participate in watching pornography? Do you still do drugs or get drunk sometimes? Are you still angry and bitter towards people? Are you living in sexual sin? Still lie to people? Cheat and steal? No one is perfect and we all got some "junk" to deal with. Wouldn't you agree?

Once you decide to wage war against your mental illness, you will have to deal with your junk aka: sin. There really is no way around it; you have to deal with your sin if you are going to be free from demons. Sin equals demons. The more sin in your life, the more demons you have. It's a spiritual law. Paul told us in Romans 6:23 that the wages of sin is death. Make sense?

If you're living a lifestyle of sin then it is most likely you are collecting demons that in turn can possibly cause sickness/disease and also could be the door opener for a mental illness to afflict you. Remember that sin equals demons.

What I personally did was I started asking the Lord what things in my life He wanted me to give up. Of course, I had to stop watching evil movies, playing really "dark" video games, partaking of sexual sin, yelling at my mother, let go of unforgiveness towards others, stop believing the voices in my head, etc.

There were a lot of things that I dealt with in my heart and God gave me the grace to be free from it. If you have decided to deal with your junk, I want to encourage you to keep working with the Lord to help you get rid of all of the junk and He will come through for you. I prayed and sought God for over one and a half years to be free from a horrible cigarette addiction and eventually He came through for me. If He has come through for me over and over again, He will also come through for you. Got it?

Another thing that I did was I wrote down everything I could think of that I needed to repent of. The list was long at first but pretty soon, it got smaller and smaller. As I grew in my prayer life, learned deliverance and repented of my sins, I got closer to God and freer from the mental torment!

STEP #4
Worship

Becoming a worshipper really helped me a lot. I learned how to worship from my heart. I would go to many worship concerts and lots of different church services to get into God's holy presence and be healed. When you worship the Lord, His presence comes and in His presence is fullness of joy, healing, deliverance and freedom.

2Corinthians 3:17
Now the Lord is the Spirit; and where the Spirit of the Lord is, there is freedom.

One of the smartest things that I can remember doing that helped me with my worship and prayer life was buying an MP3 player and downloading a bunch of good Spirit-filled worship music on it. You can find good worship music online if you need some. I would put on my MP3 player and turn up the music (and sometimes the Bible on MP3) and go on really long walks while I prayed and worshipped God.

I can't tell you how much this helped me. I highly recommend it to you. The music in the ear buds helped drown out the voices and helped me focus more on my Savior. It worked great! Maybe you should start something like this today?

STEP #5
Fighting the good fight

The foundational things I learned; reading the word, prayer, worship, repentance, etc, helped me at my next step. War against satan! I decided in my heart that I was going to cast out all of the schizophrenia demons no matter how long it took me.

Pretty much every day I would put on my ear buds, pray, worship God and command satan to come out of my mind and body. I did this almost every single day and within one year's time I was completely set free from schizophrenia. You might say, "One year? That's too long!" and I say back to you, "It took me one year, it could take you only one day, one week, one month, one year, or longer. It doesn't matter! If you have decided to become a disciple of Jesus and fight these demons, then you have to be in this for the long haul." Are you willing to keep fighting until you see freedom? I was willing and guess what, God came through for me. I am free! Don't you want to be free, too?

The kind of heart I had at the time though was this – I told God if I was never healed of schizophrenia, that I would still do my best to serve Him. Is this you today? Are you willing to still serve God if you possibly never get healed of your mental illness? Are you?

I believe that's the type of mentality you have to have if you are going to fight these demons that cause mental torment. My thought is that someone should have the mentality that they will fight until the day they see Jesus in glory, if needs be. I know you have that type of attitude in you. It's time to fight back!

STEP #6
Mentorship

Finding a mentor is a very important thing and could help you a lot. Many times the demons try to get the mentally ill person to isolate so they won't go to church, prayer meetings, Bible studies, etc. Don't listen to them anymore! Get out of bed, walk out of your house and go to church. If you can't get out of your house yet, that's ok, try to find some good teachings to listen/watch online. Find someone who preaches the message of grace, truth and love. The demons usually want people to listen to religion, legalism and hell. Don't fall for it. God isn't mad at you and wants to become your best friend. Don't take my word for it, but instead believe what God's word says.

James 2:23
Abraham believed God and He was called a friend of God.

One day at my church I met a Christian counselor that helped me through a lot of the deliverance process that I went through. I am very thankful to God for that man and his wife helping me for several years. Thank you Mike and Karen!

Many times during this period of my life, I didn't know the truth because the voices would start lying to me and my mentor could help me see things in a different light.

Without a mentor it would have been a lot harder for me. I believe you need to find a good Christian mentor who understands the battle that you are in. Pray and ask Jesus to send you someone to help you. I prayed for a long while until my mentor showed up. God always answers prayers, but not always in our timing. Be patient, He will answer. Ask God today to bring you a mentor to help disciple you. I believe that this is something that all Christians need; a mentor.

CHAPTER 4
Fighting Until You Win

I do not know everything, I can just go by what I have
been through and what I believe the Lord has shown me
about getting free. First thing is this; don't worry about
taking medications, God is not mad at you for taking
psyche medications. It is not a sin to take medications to
help you with your symptoms. It's nowhere written in the
Bible listed as a sin. Do you understand this?

Think of it this way, it's not a sin to put a bandage over
your wound, is it? The same way you can use a bandage
to cover the symptom of a wound is the same way you
can take medications to cover a symptom of a mental
illness or any other sickness. Make sense? Please stop
condemning yourself for taking medications. The devil is
telling you a lie. Don't believe him, instead tell him to
shut up and come out of your head in the name of Jesus!

The devil used to tell me that my medications were evil
and if I took them then it meant that I had no faith. It was
all a lie. I don't (and can't) give medical advice, but one
thing I can tell you about your medications is always take
them as prescribed. A lot of times I would skip days or
weeks of my medications and that messed my mind up
even worse. Please remember to always take your
medications as prescribed by a medical doctor.

What I did was once I started to feel better I worked with
my medical professional to wean off of my medications
very slowly. And guess what? One day I weaned off all
of them so much that I no longer had to take them! It was

done with my doctor and my family's help and instruction. Please don't just stop taking all of your meds. That is not good for anyone's brain chemistry or body to do that.

My point is that God is not mad at you for taking meds right now in your life. He understands what you are dealing with and if it is your desire to eventually wean off the meds, let your doctor and supporters know and they can help you through the process. I believe that is the best way to do it.

Another thing that helped me was every time the voices came to me and told me I was evil (or that I had no faith) for taking my medications, I prayed to God and told Him that I was taking the meds for my symptoms of mental illness but I was looking towards Him as my healer. Guess what? It worked! The voices of condemnation and guilt left me. Why don't you try that next time the voices attack you for taking your medications? You can overcome all voices of the enemy by your faith. All he does is lie to you. Don't you see that yet?

I am glad I covered the medication issues that tormented me for so long. I hope what I wrote here helps someone dealing with a similar issue about their medications. God loves you if you take medications or not. Either way, He loves and cares about you. That's the truth!

Now, let's move on to learn about how to get the voices and torment out of your mind. Along with repentance and learning how to worship and pray, you can also learn how to minister deliverance to yourself. But how does

someone actually cast a demon out of their own self?
Believe it or not, it really is pretty easy. I will just share
about my experience with how I have done deliverance
on myself before and maybe it will help you too.

Try to find a quiet place like a bedroom or living room.
Lie down on a bed, comfy chair or couch. Close your
eyes and start to pray to Jesus and confess all of your sins
to Him from your heart. Ask Him to come by His Spirit
and to help you overcome all of your mental torment.
Confess that you believe the word of God where it says
in the Book of Mark, Chapter 16, "these signs will follow
those who believe in My (Jesus) name; they shall cast out
demons". Then, start thanking Him for His love, grace
and mercy towards you in your life. When you are ready;
take a couple of deep breaths and then say, "satan, I
command you by the name of Jesus Christ to start
coming out of my mind, body and soul right now!" Keep
saying that to him until you possibly might feel
something releasing you or maybe moving around in
your stomach or head.

Tell the demons again and again to come out in the
mighty name of Jesus Christ! Keep telling them over and
over again until the demons start letting you go. They
come out usually by coughing, yawning, spitting, gas,
sneezing, and sometimes you will actually puke up the
demons. I know it sounds weird and crazy, but that's just
the way I have noticed evil spirits come out of people's
bodies.

Do not be afraid of demons. They are subject to you
through your faith in Jesus Christ!

Luke 10:19
Behold, I give unto you power to tread on serpents and
scorpions, and over all the power of the enemy: and
nothing shall by any means hurt you.

Luke 10:20
Nevertheless in this rejoice not, that the spirits are
subject unto you; but rather rejoice, because your names
are written in heaven.

Keep commanding satan to come out of you in the name
of Jesus Christ. Bind them (tie their power up) by the
name of Jesus Christ and cast them out of your head. You
can do it, it's not hard. Yes, it does sometimes take some
work and perseverance, but you have faith! Don't get
discouraged, keep commanding them to come out until
they manifest and start leaving your body and mind. If
some don't manifest or come out the first couple times
you minister deliverance to yourself, don't worry, just
keep going after them. They will eventually start coming
out of you, if you continue with ministering deliverance
to yourself whenever you have your prayer times. You
can also ask a spiritual mature/strong Christian friend to
help you pray and cast out your demons as well.

There are resources on the Internet and at some Christian
bookstores to read and learn about casting out demons.
You can also go to my ministry's website at
www.TheFathersFriends.org and get help through some
of our ministry resources too. I am not the only one who
knows about deliverance, many people have written
books on the subject. If you use an online search engine,
try searching keywords like "deliverance", "deliverance

books", "casting out demons", "deliverance teachings", "how to cast out demons", etc. I recommend learning as much as you can about deliverance if you are going to wage war against mental illness.

I have learned a lot about demons and deliverance and a couple of things I found that really help in this battle is to have a repentant heart and to command satan to come out in Jesus name. No need to have conversations with demons (like you might see on the Internet or television) or interact with them in anyway. Tell them to shut up and come out. If you are wanting to serve Jesus, have a repentant heart and commanding satan to come out, I believe the demons will start leaving your body and mind and eventually they will be gone in Jesus name!

I believe some of the reasons he is allowed to stay attached to an individual is because of a lie that the person is currently believing, unconfessed sin, generational curses, unforgivesness, etc. Untangle the lies, confess your sins to God, forgive others, and get those demons out!

One thing I do want to clear up for a moment is this. Please remember that just because someone is a Christian and has demons, doesn't mean that they are not saved and not on their way to heaven. They are still saved and get to go to heaven because of their belief in Jesus Christ's finished work on the cross!

Believe it or not, I believe that everyone has to deal with their demons; most people just don't know that they have demons and they live with them in ignorance. You are not a bad person if you have demons and are still a Christian. God loves you and wants to show you the truth that you can be free from the tormentors through Jesus' name!

If you are a born again Christian, the demons are not in your spirit man, but in your body, soul, or mind. Every born again believer no matter how many demons they have will end up going to heaven when they die.

Stop worrying; you haven't lost your salvation if you possibly have demons tormenting you. It's ok; God still loves and accepts you just the way that you are. He is so kind and good, He is your heavenly Father. I used to be worried about the above issue and that is why I added this part into this book. It is to calm your fears that you might have lost your salvation because you have demons. You haven't lost your salvation. God is still with you and always will be. Be encouraged today that the Holy Spirit wants to completely set you free!

Keep doing deliverance on yourself as long as you have to. It took me doing deliverance for many months, pretty much every day to deal with some of the strongholds that I picked up in my mind. It's ok though, just keep fighting and victory will come. Keep seeking Jesus, repenting and casting out your demons. It is biblical and it actually really does work. Once you have overcome your own demons, you will have authority and power to help others cast out their demons!

CHAPTER 5
Defeating Lies With Truth

I believe that one of the most major reasons people with
mental illnesses sometimes take a while to be free is
because many of them have been "conditioned" by satan
to believe his lies. Sometimes it takes a while to
overcome specific lies. For instance, I used to believe
everyone hated me (spirit of rejection). I battled this
thing for a long period of time. But through that long
battle, I gained many valuable insights to help others be
free from that specific tormenting spirit. Remember that
in Romans Chapter 8 it says that "all things work
together for good for those who love God and who are
called according to His purposes."

It helped me to write down every lie that I was believing
about myself, others and God. For instance, I wrote down
things like "I am going to hell" or "I am ugly" or "I will
never be married". I wrote down all the lies. After I wrote
down all the lies, I then went through the Bible and found
all the scriptures that defeated those particular lies. In
Chapter 4 of the Book of Hebrews it says that "the word
of God is sharper than any two edged sword." It is the
greatest weapon to defeat the lies of satan. The word
works!

After finding the verse(s) that dealt with a specific lie, I
then would renounce the lie and speak the truth from
what was written in the Bible. I would do that over and
over until the lies were destroyed. This is one way to pull
down a stronghold; beating the lie with the truth.

For some people, it might take longer than others to defeat certain lies because some lies have been ingrained in us since we were little children. For instance, you might believe some lie that your mother told you when you were five years old. You might have lived with that lie in your head that was from your mother until you were 50+ years old. See how it sometimes takes a little longer to defeat the bigger strongholds? That's ok though; you stick this out and you will see victory in Jesus name!

The enemy attacks your mind like he is throwing an arrow into your head. If one of the arrows (lies) gets into your head and you receive it as truth, then he throws a couple more arrows (lies) into your head. Receiving lies is actually a sin (because it's opposite of God's truth) and allows the enemy an inroad to torment you. Stop receiving the lies and speak the truth instead. What could happen if you keep believing lies from satan is that you could have a lot of lies in your head and that usually leads to more strongholds of the enemy in your mind. This could then eventually lead to more torment for you. I hope you are getting this here?

I believe one major key to victory is to catch the lies when they first hit your thoughts and do your best to take it "captive" like Paul said in the below passage.

<u>2Corinthians 10:3-6</u>
For though we walk in the flesh, we do not war after the flesh: (For the weapons of our warfare are not carnal, but mighty through God to the pulling down of strong holds;) Casting down imaginations, and every high thing

that exalteth itself against the knowledge of God, and bringing into captivity every thought to the obedience of Christ; And having in a readiness to revenge all disobedience, when your obedience is fulfilled.

See, Paul knew how to deal with these types of things too. I hope you move forward to demolish the strongholds with truth, reject the lies, catch the arrows and not receive lies from satan any longer. It takes some time to learn how to defeat your own demons, but through your journey of defeating mental illness strongholds, I believe you will learn some great things that will help others overcome as well. I truly believe you are called to become a powerfully anointed spiritual warrior!

CONCLUSION

You are not your diagnosis. You are a beloved child of
God that is about to be set free by the power of the Holy
Spirit. I honestly believe that mental illness is not
"incurable" as many people say it is. I am living proof
that you can be delivered and healed. Be encouraged
today that life is not hopeless and you have great value to
Father God. Please remember to keep fighting until you
win. Never give up because God has a great destiny for
you. Fight! Fight! Fight!

My Prayer for you

"Father God, I pray for the person reading this right now,
I pray that the revelation that they can be set free from
mental illness enlightens them. God, as someone who has
personally overcome schizophrenia by faith in You, I ask
that the same courage, faith and strength that You gave
me be given to this person. I pray the anointing of the
Holy Spirit rest upon them as they decide to head down
the Narrow Road with Jesus, deal with their junk, grow
in their prayer life, worship Jesus and drive out all of
their evil spirits. Help them to never give up, but to
pursue You with everything they have. I ask that You
find them a good Christian mentor, someone who will
help them through this time in their life, but most of all, I
pray that they grow extremely close to the Holy Spirit
through this experience. Please remind them every day
that they are not alone in this battle, but that You are their
shield, defender, refuge, healer and deliverer. Thank you
for loving the mentally ill, Lord Jesus, amen."

I HATE THE DEVIL
Audio CD

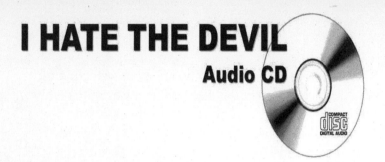

Hear Nick Griemsmann's amazing testimony of being healed of an "incurable" mental illness called schizophrenia. This audio teaching can also help you start your deliverance process, receive healing and it also includes a prayer time to help you receive the baptism of the Holy Spirit. Download the I Hate The Devil cd for No-Charge today! Also available in Spanish.

www.TheFathersFriends.org

Most *Griemsmann Media* products are available at special quantity discounts for bulk purchases for fund-raising, educational needs, churches, libraries, bookstores, etc. Please contact us for more information.

Griemsmann Media
P.O. Box 60065
Phoenix, Arizona 85082
www.GriemsmannMedia.com